Hand Bone Age

Vicente Gilsanz • Osman Ratib

Hand Bone Age

A Digital Atlas of Skeletal Maturity

Second Edition

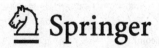

Prof. Vicente Gilsanz
Department of Radiology
Childrens Hospital Los Angeles
4650 Sunset Blvd., MS#81
Los Angeles, CA 90027
USA

Prof. Osman Ratib
University Hospital of Geneva
Nuclear Medicine Division
24, Rue Micheli-du-Crest
1205 Geneva
Switzerland

ISBN 978-3-642-23761-4   e-ISBN 978-3-642-23762-1
DOI 10.1007/978-3-642-23762-1
Springer Heidelberg Dordrecht London New York

Library of Congress Control Number: 2011940860

Springer is part of Springer Science+Business Media (www.springer.com)

Acknowledgement

This atlas would not have been possible without the exceptional contributions of Doctors Maria Ines Boechat und Xiaodong Liu, who painstakingly helped in the review, interpretation and assessment of hundreds of hand and wrist radiographs.

Contents

Introduction

Bone age assessment is frequently performed in pediatric patients to evaluate growth and to diagnose and manage a multitude of endocrine disorders and pediatric syndromes. For decades, the determination of bone maturity has relied on a visual evaluation of the skeletal development of the hand and wrist, most commonly using the Greulich and Pyle atlas. With the advent of digital imaging, multiple attempts have been made to develop image-processing techniques that automatically extract the key morphological features of ossification in the bones to provide a more effective and objective approach to skeletal maturity assessments. However, the design of computer algorithms capable of automatically rendering bone age has been impeded by the complexity of evaluating the wide variations in bone mineralization tempo, shape and size encompassed in the large number of ossification centers in the hand and wrist. Clearly, developing an accurate digital reference that integrates the quantitative morphological traits associated with the different degrees of skeletal maturation of 21 tubular bones in the hand and 8 carpal bones in the wrist is not an easy task.

In the development of this digital atlas, we circumvented the difficulties associated with the design of software that integrates all morphological parameters through the selection of an alternative approach: the creation of artificial, idealized, sex- and age-specific images of skeletal development. The models were generated through rigorous analyses of the maturation of each ossification center in the hands and wrists of healthy children, and the construction of virtual images that incorporate composites of the average development for each ossification center in each age group. This computer-generated set of images should serve as a practical alternative to the reference books currently available.

V. Gilsanz and O. Ratib, *Hand Bone Age*,
DOI 10.1007/978-3-642-23762-1_1, © Springer-Verlag Berlin Heidelberg 2012

Bone Development

2

Skeletal maturity is a measure of development incorporating the size, shape and degree of mineralization of bone to define its proximity to full maturity. The assessment of skeletal maturity involves a rigorous examination of multiple factors and a fundamental knowledge of the various processes by which bone develops.

Longitudinal growth in the long bones of the extremities occurs through the process of endochondral ossification. In contrast, the width of the bones increases by development of skeletal tissue directly from fibrous membrane. The latter is the mechanism by which ossification of the calvarium, the flat bones of the pelvis, the scapulae, and the body of the mandible occurs. Initial calcification begins near the center of the shaft of long bones in a region called the primary ossification center [1].

Although many flat bones, including the carpal bones, ossify entirely from this primary center, all of the long bones develop secondary centers that appear in the cartilage of the extremities of the bone. Maturation in these centers proceeds in a manner identical to that in the primary centers with ossification of cartilage and invasion of osteoclasts and osteoblasts. The bone ossified from the primary center is the diaphysis, while the bone ossified from the secondary center is the epiphysis. As the secondary center is progressively ossified, the cartilage is replaced by bone until only a thin layer of cartilage, the epiphyseal plate, separates the diaphyseal bone from the epiphysis. The part of the diaphysis that abuts on the epiphysis is referred to as the metaphysis and represents the growing end of the bone. As long as the epiphyseal cartilage plate persists, both the diaphysis and epiphysis continue to grow, but, eventually, the osteoblasts cease to multiply and the epiphyseal plate is ossified. At that time, the osseous structures of the diaphysis and epiphysis are fused and growth ceases [1] (Fig. 2.1).

In the fetal phase of life, the principle interest in skeletal growth is associated with the diagnosis of prematurity. The end of the embryonic period and the beginning of the fetus is marked by the event of calcification, which begins at 8 or 9 weeks. By the 13th fetal week, most primary centers of the tubular bones are well-developed into diaphyses, and, at birth, all diaphyses are completely ossified, while most of the epiphyses are still cartilaginous. Ossification of the distal femoral epiphysis

V. Gilsanz and O. Ratib, *Hand Bone Age*,
DOI 10.1007/978-3-642-23762-1_2, © Springer-Verlag Berlin Heidelberg 2012

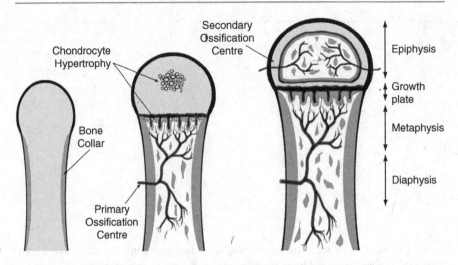

Fig. 2.1 Schematic representation of endochondral bone formation. Skeletal maturity is mainly assessed by the degree of development and ossification of the secondary ossification centers in the epiphysis

begins during the last 2 months of gestation, and this secondary center is present in most full term babies. Similarly, the ossification center for the proximal epiphysis of the humerus usually appears about the 40th week of gestation. On the other hand, the centers for the proximal epiphyses of the femur and tibia may not be present in full term infants, but appear in the first few months of life [2, 3].

After birth, the epiphyses gradually ossify in a largely predictable order, and, at skeletal maturity, fuse with the main body of the bone. Comparing the degree of maturation of the epiphyses to normal age-related standards forms the basis for the assessment of skeletal maturity, the measure of which is commonly called "bone age" or "skeletal age". It is not clear which factors determine a normal maturational pattern, but it is certain that genetics, environmental factors, and hormones, such as thyroxine, growth hormone, and sex steroids, play important roles. Studies in patients with mutations of the gene for the estrogen receptor or for aromatase enzyme have demonstrated that it is estrogen that is primarily responsible for ultimate epiphyseal fusion, although it seems unlikely that estrogen alone is responsible for all skeletal maturation [4].

Clinical Applications for Skeletal Determinations

A single reading of skeletal age informs the clinician of the relative maturity of a patient at a particular time in his or her life, and, integrated with other clinical findings, separates the normal from the relatively advanced or re tarded. Successive skeletal age readings indicate the direction of the child's development and/or show his or her progress under treatment. In normal subjects, bone age should be roughly within 10% of the chronological age. Greater discordance between skeletal age and chronological age occurs in children who are obese or who start puberty early, as their skeletal age is accelerated.

There are two main applications for evaluations of skeletal maturation: the diagnosis of growth disorders and the prediction of final adult height.

Diagnosis of Growth Disorders

Assessments of skeletal age are of great importance for the diagnosis of growth disorders, which may be classified into two broad categories with different etiologies, prognoses and treatments. Primary growth deficiency is due to an intrinsic defect in the skeletal system, such as bone dysplasia, resulting from either a genetic defect or prenatal damage and leading to shortening of the diaphysis without significant delay of epiphyseal maturation. Hence, in this form of growth disorder, the potential normal bone growth (and therefore, body growth) is impaired, while skeletal age is not delayed or is delayed much less than is height.

Secondary growth deficiency is related to factors, generally outside the skeletal system, that impair epiphyseal or osseous maturation. These factors may be nutritional, metabolic, or unknown, as in the syndrome of idiopathic (constitutional) growth delay. In this form of growth retardation, skeletal age and height may be delayed to nearly the same degree, but, with treatment, the potential exists for reaching normal adult height.

The distinction between these categories may be difficult in some instances in which skeletal age is delayed to a lesser degree than height. In general, however, differentiation between primary and secondary categories of growth failure can be determined from clinical findings and skeletal age [5].

Final Height Predictions

The adult height of a child who grows up under favorable environmental circumstances is, to a large extent, dependent on heredity. The final height of the child may, therefore, be postulated from parental heights. Indeed, various methods of final height predictions, which take into account parental height, have been described [6]. A child's adult height can also be predicted from his or her heights at earlier ages, with correlations on the order of 0.8. However, children differ greatly in rate of development; some attain maturity at a relatively early age, while others have a slow tempo and finish growing relatively late. Hence, knowledge of the degree of development increases the accuracy of final height predictions. The only practical guide to acquire this knowledge is by assessment of skeletal maturity, usually estimated from a hand and wrist radiograph.

Tables for prediction of ultimate height based on the individual's height, skeletal age, sex, age, and growth rate have been published. Using skeletal age for prediction of ultimate height, it is also possible to make a rough calculation as follows: measure the individual's height, plot it on a standard growth curve, and extrapolate the value horizontally to the age on the chart that is equal to the bone age. If the point of extrapolation falls between the 5th and 95th centiles, then a guarded prediction of normal adult stature can be given. The closer the extrapolated value is to the 50th centile, the more accurate it is likely to be [5].

Other bone age and height prediction methods commonly in use are those of Bayley-Pinneau, Roche et al. and Tanner-Whitehouse [7–9]. All of these methods use radiographs of the hand and wrist to assess skeletal maturity and were based on population data from normal children followed to adult height. Overall, these methods have 95% confidence intervals of 7–9 cm when used to predict the final height of individuals. It is necessary to realize, however, that estimations of final height are most accurate in children who are healthy, and, in the sick, these predictions are less reliable.

Below is the formula for the prediction of adult height estimated by J.M. Tanner et al. [9]:

$$Predicted\ Final\ Height = Height\ Coefficient \times Present\ Height\ (cm)\ +$$
$$Age\ Coefficient \times Chronological\ Age\ (years) +$$
$$Bone\ Age\ Coefficient \times Bone\ Age\ (years) +$$
$$Constant$$

In girls, these investigators incorporated knowledge of whether or not menarche had occurred, which improved their predictions. The tables for the coefficients for prediction of adult height are on pages 93 and 94.

Conventional Techniques for Skeletal Determinations

In the evaluation of physical development in children, variations in maturation rate are poorly described by chronological age. Thus, for many decades, scientists have sought better techniques to assess the degree of development from birth to full maturity. Measures of height, weight, and body mass, although closely related to biological maturation, are not sufficiently accurate due to the wide variations in body size. Similarly, the large varia tions in dental development have prevented the use of dental age as an overall measure of maturation, and other clinically established techniques are of limited value. As examples, the age at menarche, although an important biological indicator, relates to only half the population, and determinations of sexual development using the Tanner classification, while an extremely useful clinical tool, is subjective and restricted to the adolescent period. Unfortunately, most available maturational "age" scales have specific uses and tempos that do not necessarily coincide.

Skeletal age, or bone age, the most common measure for biological maturation of the growing human, derives from the examination of successive stages of skeletal development, as viewed in hand-wrist radiographs. This technique, used by pediatricians, orthopedic surgeons, physical anthropologists and all those interested in the study of human growth, is currently the only available indicator of

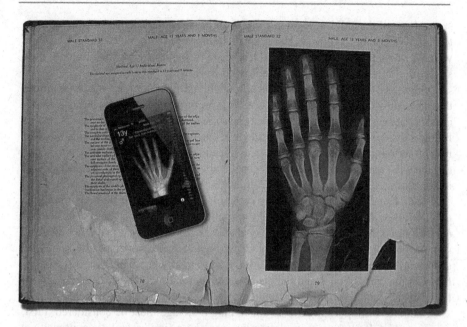

Fig. 2.2 Comparison of the traditional Greulich and Pyle atlas used for determination of bone maturity from hand radiographs and the electronic alternative, a digital atlas of "idealized" hand radiographs that can be reviewed on standard hand-held PDAs

development that spans the entire growth period, from birth to maturity. Essentially, the degree of skeletal maturity depends on two features: growth of the area undergoing ossification, and deposition of calcium in that area. While these two traits may not keep pace with each other, nor are they always present concurrently, they follow a fairly definite pattern and time schedule, from infancy to adulthood. Through radiographs, this process provides a valuable criterion for estimating normal and abnormal growth and maturation (Fig. 2.2).

Greulich and Pyle and Tanner-Whitehouse (TW2) are the most prevalently employed skeletal age techniques today [10, 11]. Despite their differing theoretical approaches, both are based on the recognition of maturity indicators, i.e., changes in the radiographic appearance of the epiphyses of tubular bones from the earliest stages of ossification until fusion with the diaphysis, or changes in flat bones until attainment of adult shape [12].

The standards established by Greulich and Pyle, undoubtedly the most popular method, consist of two series of standard plates obtained from hand-wrist radiographs of white, upper middle-class boys and girls enrolled in the Brush Foundation Growth Study from 1931 to 1942. Represented in the Greulich and Pyle atlas are 'central tendencies', which are modal levels of maturity within chronological age groups. The skeletal age assigned to each standard corresponds to the age of the children on whom the standard was based. When using the Greulich and Pyle method, the radiograph to be assessed is compared with the series of standard plates, and the age given to the standard plate that fits most closely is assigned as the skeletal age of the child. It is often convenient to interpolate between two standards to assign a suitable age to a radiograph. The apparent simplicity and speed with which a skeletal age can be assigned has made this atlas the most commonly used standard of reference for skeletal maturation worldwide.

Underlying the construction of the Greulich and Pyle atlas are the assumptions that, in healthy children, skeletal maturation is uniform, that all bones have an identical skeletal age, and that the appearance and subsequent development of body centers follow a fixed pattern. However, considerable evidence suggests that a wide range of normal variation exists in the pattern of ossification of the different bones of the hand and the wrist and that this variation is genetically determined. In fact, most standards in the atlas include bones that differ considerably in their levels of maturity [10].

Greulich and Pyle did not formally recommend any specific technique for the use of their atlas. Rather, they suggested that atlas users develop their own method depending on their preferences. Pyle et al. did, however, suggest the rather cumbersome approach that each ossification center be assigned a bone-specific bone age, and the average of the ages calculated. By and large, when there is a discrepancy between the carpal bones and the distal centers, greater weight should be assigned to the distal centers because they tend to correlate better with growth potential [5].

A number of important caveats concerning bone age must be considered. First, experience in skeletal maturity determinations and a similar analytic approach are essential to enhance inter- and intra-observer reproducibility. Clinical studies and trials involving bone age as an outcome measure greatly benefit from the inclusion of experienced readers who use similar approaches in their assessments. Second, the normal rate of skeletal matura tion differs between males and females, and ethnic variability exists. Lastly, these references are not necessarily applicable to children with skeletal dysplasias, endocrine abnormalities or a variety of other causes of growth retardation.

Computer Assisted Techniques for Skeletal Determinations

With the advent of digital imaging, several investigators have attempted to provide an objective computer-assisted measure for bone age determinations and have developed image processing techniques from reference databases of normal children that automatically extract key features of hand radiographs [13–17]. To date, however, attempts to develop automated image analysis techniques capable of extracting quantitative measures of the morphological traits depicting skeletal maturity have been hindered by the inability to account for the great variability in development and ossification of the multiple bones in the hand and wrist. In an attempt to overcome these difficulties, automated techniques are being developed that primarily rely on measures of a few ossification centers, such as those of the epiphyses.

In the design of this digital atlas, the complexities associated with the design of software that integrates all morphological parameters was circumvented through the selection of an alternative approach. We designed artificial, idealized, sex- and age-specific images of skeletal development that incorporated the different degrees of maturation of each ossification center in the hand and wrist. The idealized image was derived from a composite of several hand radiographs from healthy children and adolescents that were identified as the perfect average for each ossification center in each age group.

Our aim was to provide a portable alternative to the reference books currently available, while avoiding the complexity of computer assisted image analysis. The wide adoption of personal digital assistants (PDAs) and pocket computer devices allowed the implementation of a low-cost portable solution that could effectively replace the traditional reference books. Technical challenges included the development of proper compression and image enhancement techniques for interpretation of hand radiographs on a small screen with adequate quality, and the need to store a large number of images on instruments with limited memory capacity.

Indicators of Skeletal Maturity in Children and Adolescents

3

The purpose of this section is to describe which bones in the hand and wrist are the most suitable indicators of skeletal maturity during the different phases of postnatal development. In the majority of healthy children, there is an established sequence of ossification for the carpal (Fig. 3.1), metacarpal and phalangeal bones, which is remarkably constant and the same for both sexes. Overall, the first ossification center to appear in hand and wrist radiographs is the capitate, and the last is, most often, the sesamoid of the adductor pollicis of the thumb [18].

The first epiphyseal center to appear is that of the distal radius, followed by those of the proximal phalanges, the metacarpals, the middle phalanges, the distal phalanges, and, finally, the ulna. There are, however, two main exceptions to this sequence: the epiphysis of the distal phalanx of the thumb commonly appears at the same time as the epiphyses of the metacarpals, and the epiphysis of the middle phalanx of the fifth finger is frequently the last to ossify.

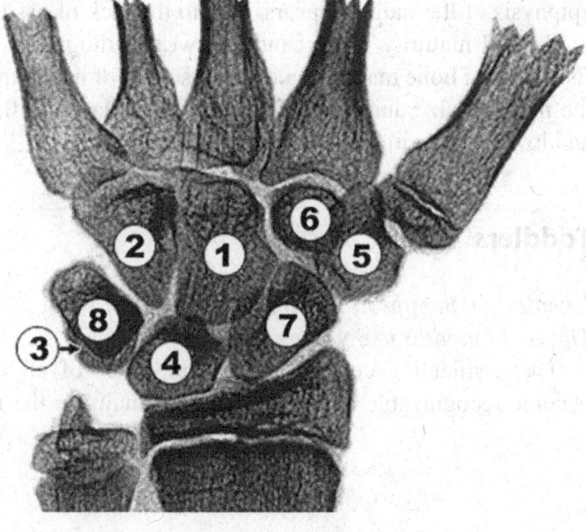

Fig. 3.1 Depiction of the order of appearance of the individual carpal bones. The usual sequence is: capitate *1*, hamate *2*, triquetral *3*, lunate *4*, trapezium *5*, trapezoid *6*, navicular or scaphoid *7* and pisiform *8*. The distal epiphysis of the radius ossifies before the triquetum and that of the ulna before the pisiform

V. Gilsanz and O. Ratib, *Hand Bone Age*,
DOI 10.1007/978-3-642-23762-1_3, © Springer-Verlag Berlin Heidelberg 2012

Since the predictive value of the ossification centers differs and changes during growth, the reviewer should primarily focus on the centers that best characterize skeletal development for the subject's chronological age. To facilitate bone age assessments, we have divided skeletal development into six major categories and highlighted in parentheses the specific ossification centers that are the best predictors of skeletal maturity for each group:

1. Infancy (the carpal bones and radial epiphyses);
2. Toddlers (the number of epiphyses visible in the long bones of the hand);
3. Pre-puberty (the size of the phalangeal epiphyses);
4. Early and Mid-puberty (the size of the phalangeal epiphyses);
5. Late Puberty (the degree of epiphyseal fusion); and,
6. Post-puberty (the degree of epiphyseal fusion of the radius and ulna).

While these divisions are arbitrary, we chose stages that reflect pubertal status, since osseous development conforms better with the degree of sexual development than with the chronologic age. The features that characterize these successive stages of skeletal development are outlined in schematic drawings depicting their appearance as seen in posterior anterior roentgenograms of the hand and wrist.

Infancy

Females: Birth to 10 months of age
Males: Birth to 14 months of age

All carpal bones and all epiphyses in the phalanges, metacarpals, radius and ulna lack ossification in the full-term newborn. The ossification centers of the capitate and hamate become apparent at about 3 months of age and remain the only useful observable features for the next 6 months. At about 10 months of age for girls, and about 1 year and 3 months of age for boys, a small center of ossification in the distal epiphysis of the radius appears. Due to the lack of ossification centers, assessment of skeletal maturity using hand and wrist radiographs during infancy is difficult. Estimates of bone maturation in the first year of life frequently require evaluation of the number, size and configuration of secondary ossification centers in the upper and lower extremities (Fig. 3.2).

Toddlers

Females: 10 months to 2 years of age
Males: 14 months to 3 years of age

The ossification centers for the epiphyses of all phalanges and metacarpals become recognizable during this stage, usually in the middle finger first, and the

Fig. 3.2 During infancy,
bone age is primarily based
on the presence or absence of
ossification of the capitate,
the hamate and the distal
epiphysis of the radius. The
capitate usually appears
slightly earlier than the
hamate, and has a larger
ossification center and
rounder shape. The distal
radial epiphysis appears later

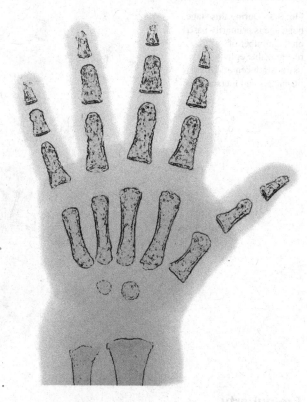

fifth finger last. Bone age determinations are primarily based on the assessment of
the number of identifiable epiphyseal ossification centers, which generally appear in
an orderly characteristic pattern, as follows:
1. Epiphyses of the proximal phalanges;
2. Epiphyses of the metacarpals;
3. Epiphyses of the middle phalanges; and,
4. Epiphyses of the distal phalanges.
   Two common exceptions to this rule are:
1. The early appearance of the ossification center of the distal phalanx of the thumb,
   which is usually recognizable at 1 year and 3 months in males, and 1 year and 6
   months in females (Fig. 3.3); and,
2. The late appearance of the ossification center of the middle phalanx of the fifth
   finger, which is the last phalangeal epiphysis to appear.
   The number and degree of maturation of the carpal bones in the wrist are less
useful indicators at this stage, as only three or four (capitate, hamate and lunate and,
at times, trapezoid) are recognizable.

Fig. 3.3 During this stage, bone age is primarily based on the number of recognizable epiphyseal ossification centers in the phalanges and metacarpals

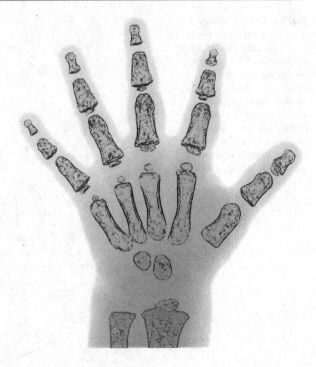

Pre-puberty

Females: 2 years to 7 years of age
Males: 3 years to 9 years of age

Assessments of skeletal maturity in pre-pubertal children are primarily based on the epiphyseal size of the phalanges as they relate to the adjacent metaphyses. During this stage of development, the ossification centers for the epiphyses increase in width and thickness, and eventually assume a transverse diameter as wide as the metaphyses. More weight is given to the size of the epiphyses in the distal phalanges than to that in the middle phalanges, and even less to that in the proximal phalanges. However, since the development of the distal phalanges appears similar at several different ages, at times the assessment is also based on the degree of maturity for the epiphyses of the middle phalanges. On very rare occasions when there continues to be doubt, the development of the proximal phalanx may be included in the assessment (Figs. 3.4 and 3.5).

The epiphysis of the ulna and all carpal bones, with the exception of the pisiform, usually become recognizable before puberty. However, these ossification centers, like those of the metacarpals, are less reliable indicators of bone age at this stage of life.

Fig. 3.4 Depiction of the progressive growth of the width of the epiphyses, which, during this stage of development, become as wide as the metaphyses

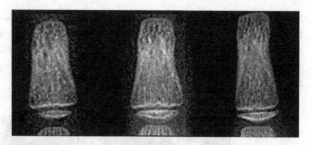

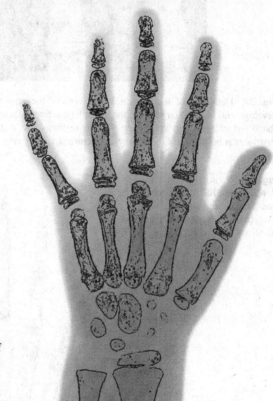

Fig. 3.5 Assessments of bone age are primarily based on the degree of difference in width between the smaller epiphyses and the larger metaphyses at the distal and middle phalanges

Early and Mid-puberty

Females: 7 years to 13 years of age
Males: 9 years to 14 years of age

As in pre-pubertal children, assessments of skeletal maturity in early and mid-puberty are also based on the size of the epiphyses in the distal phalanges (first) and the middle phalanges (second). The epiphyses at this stage continue to grow and their widths become greater than the metaphyses. Thereafter, the contours of the epiphyses begin to overlap, or cap, the metaphyses. This capping effect is depicted in a two-dimensional radiograph as small bony outgrowths, like tiny horns, on both sides of the shaft (Figs. 3.6 and 3.7).

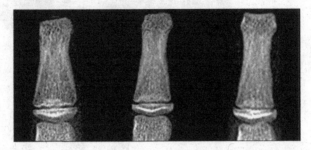

Fig. 3.6 Depiction of the progressive growth of the epiphyses, which, during this stage of development, become larger than the metaphyses. Special attention is also placed on epiphyseal shape, which, prior to epiphyseal fusion, overlaps the metaphyses, depicting tiny horn-like structures at both ends of the epiphysis (picture at *far-right*)

Fig. 3.7 During this stage of development, like for prepubertal and late-pubertal children, assessments are based primarily on the distal and middle phalanges

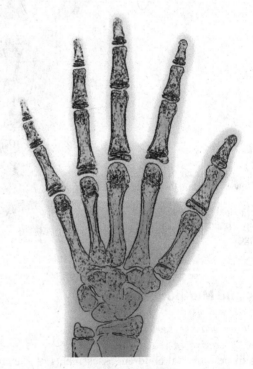

The pisiform and the sesamoid in the tendon of the abductor pollicis, just medial to the head of the first metacarpal, become recognizable during puberty. However, these centers, as well as those of the other carpals and metacarpals, are less reliable as indicators of bone age at this stage of development.

Late Puberty

Females: 13 years to 15 years of age
Males: 14 years to 16 years of age

Assessments of skeletal maturity in this stage are primarily based on the degree of epiphyseal fusion of the distal phalanges. Fusion of the epiphyses to the metaphyses in the long bones of the hand tends to occur in an orderly characteristic pattern, as follows:

1. Fusion of the distal phalanges;
2. Fusion of the metacarpals;
3. Fusion of the proximal phalanges; and,
4. Fusion of the middle phalanges.

Because of their morphologies, the epiphyseal fusion of the metacarpals is poorly depicted by radiographs and greater attention is, therefore, placed on the degree of fusion at the phalanges. Since all carpal bones have now attained their early adult shape, they are of less value for determination of bone age (Figs. 3.8 and 3.9).

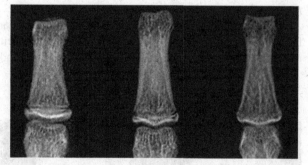

Fig. 3.8 Depiction, from left to right, of the progressive degrees of fusion of the epiphyses to the metaphyses, which usually begins at the center of the physis

Fig. 3.9 Assessments in late stages
of puberty and sexual maturity are
based on the degree of epiphyseal
fusion of the distal phalanges (*first*)
and on the degree of fusion of the
middle phalanges (*second*)

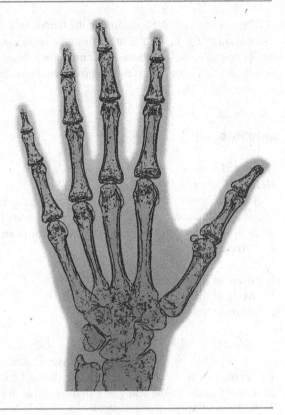

Post-puberty

Females: 15 years to 17 years of age
Males: 17 years to 19 years of age

At this stage, all carpals, metacarpals and phalanges are completely developed,
their physes are closed, and assessments of skeletal maturity are based on the degree
of epiphyseal fusion of the ulna and radius (Figs. 3.10 and 3.11).

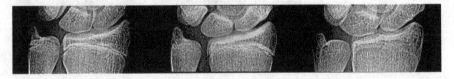

Fig. 3.10 Depiction, from left to right, of the progressive degrees of fusion of the ulna and the
radial epiphyses, which usually begins at the center of the physis

Fig. 3.11 At this stage of development, skeletal maturity is based on epiphyseal fusion of the ulna, which occurs first, and the radius

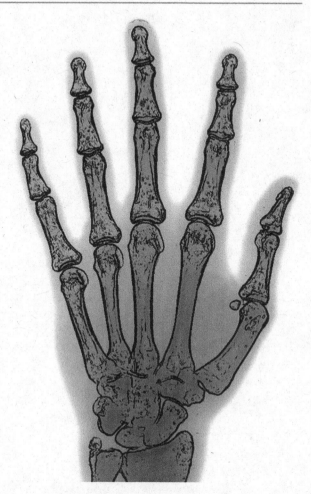

Digital Bone Age Atlas

4

Subjects

During the past two decades, multiple studies on normal growth and skeletal development have been conducted at Childrens Hospital Los Angeles. The hand and wrist radiographs obtained for these studies form the basis of the data used to develop the digital bone age atlas. Participants were healthy children and adolescents who were recruited from schools and boys and girls clubs in the Los Angeles area. All studies were approved by the local IRB and all subjects and/or their parents signed informed consent.

The hand and wrist radiographs selected as standards for the digital atlas were obtained from children whose parents and both sets of grandparents were of European descent, who had no diagnosis of chronic illness, and who were not taking any medications regularly. The height and weight of each child was between the 3rd and 97th percentiles and the Tanner stage was within 2 SD for the mean age-adjusted values [19, 20].

A total of 522 left hand and wrist radiographs were evaluated (50% female, 50% male) and were the basis for the reference standards. The standards were grouped by age based on the variability for skeletal age at the different stages of development. The intervals between groupings are roughly equal to one standard deviation for skeletal maturity at that chronological age (Table 4, page 95) and increase from 2 months in infancy to 1 year by 6 years of age. Each of the standards was selected from nine radiographs of children of the same sex and age.

Methods and Techniques

Idealized images were developed from 522 left hand and wrist radiographs of Caucasian boys and girls that were divided into 29 age groups ranging from 8 months to 18 years of age. For each age group, nine images were sorted by two independent radiologists based on the degree of skeletal maturity at different ossification centers.

V. Gilsanz and O. Ratib, *Hand Bone Age*,
DOI 10.1007/978-3-642-23762-1_4, © Springer-Verlag Berlin Heidelberg 2012

The middle image was then identified as the "average" image; half of the remaining images depicted less skeletal maturity and half depicted more skeletal maturity at the region examined. This process was applied to six different anatomical regions of the hand and wrist: the proximal, middle and distal phalanges, the metacarpals, the carpals, and, lastly, the distal radius and ulna. Frequently, the selected "middle" images for the six anatomical regions belonged to different children from the same sex and age groups. Computer image combinations allowed the merger of the different average images into one single representative idealized image for that age group.

For each age group, prior to creating a composite idealized image from the different selected key images, three image processing steps and enhancements were applied for standardization. First, the background was replaced by a uniform black setting and the image size was adjusted to fit into square images of 800×800 pixels. Second, contrast and intensity were optimized using predefined window and level thresholds. Lastly, the image was processed through a special edge enhancement filter based on an unsharp masking algorithm tailored to provide optimum sharpness of bone structure for hand-held devices.

After proper processing and enhancement, the selected images were combined to generate a single "idealized" image for each age group and for each gender. Several images, ranging from two to six, were combined by carefully replacing segments of bones through translation, rotation and warping operations to match the underlying combination image (Fig. 4.1). The result was a single image representing a combination of parts of hand radiographs from several images. Prior to using this computer-generated image as a reference, it was reviewed by two experienced pediatric radiologists to evaluate its congruency with other reference images in the digital atlas and its compliance with existing knowledge of progression of bone maturation (Figs. 4.1–4.3).

Validation of Standards and Technique

Readings of skeletal maturity using the digital atlas program were validated through comparisons of skeletal maturation determinations using the Greulich and Pyle method by two experienced radiologists. Images from an additional 200 healthy Caucasian children (100 boys, 100 girls) were examined in a double blind reading. Regardless of the radiologist or the method employed to assess skeletal maturity, strong correlations were present between chronological age and bone age, with no statistical difference observed between the digital and Greulich and Pyle atlases (Table 4.1).

An independent comparative study performed at Children's National Medical Center, in Washington DC [21], seven pediatric radiologists (mean years in practice: 14.7 years, range: 4–32 years) and five pediatric endocrinologists (mean years in practice: 11.2, range: 2–27 years) read 16 randomly selected radiographs (8 boys, 8 girls), using both the GP and the Gilsanz-Ratib (GR) digital atlas. Two electronic files of these images were created and distributed to all endocrinologists and radiologists; the only information provided was the age and sex of the patient. The first file was to

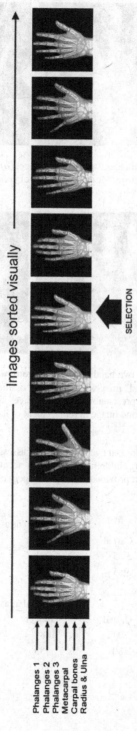

Phalanges 1
Phalanges 2
Phalanges 3
Metacarpal
Carpal bones
Radius & Ulna

Images sorted visually

SELECTION

Fig. 4.1 Method of selection of the "average" image from a set of nine normal hand radiographs of a given age group. The images were sorted by skeletal maturity six consecutive times based on six anatomical regions. Each time, the middle image was noted as the "average" image for a given anatomical region for that particular age group. This often resulted in the selection of more than one and up to six different images for a given group. An idealized "average" image was then generated by combination of the selected images. Phalanges 1, 2 and 3 indicate proximal, middle and distal, respectively

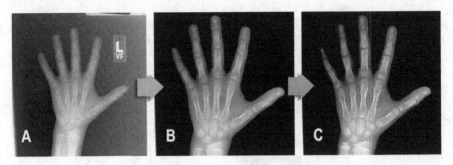

Fig. 4.2 Processing and enhancement of images. (**a**) Original image; (**b**) Background replaced by a uniform black setting and image size adjusted; (**c**) Optimization of contrast and intensity

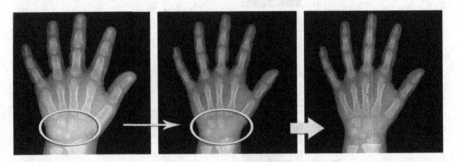

Fig. 4.3 Example of the combination of two hand radiographs from two different individuals of the same age group into a single "idealized" image. The degree of ossification of the carpal bones of the first image were selected as more representative of the "average" skeletal maturation for this age group and were transferred to the second image in replacement of its original carpal bones

Table 4.1 Correlations between chronological age and bone age assessed with the Greulich and Pyle method and the digital atlas in healthy children of European descent of all ages and in adolescents 12–15 years old. The digital system provided slightly stronger correlations, although these differences were not statistically significant

Ages 0–18 year				
	Greulich and Pyle		Digital atlas	
Sex (n)	Finger	Carpal	Finger	Carpal
Boys (100)	.987	.985	.991	.988
Girls (100)	.984	.985	.988	.987
Ages 12–15 year				
	Greulich and Pyle		Digital atlas	
Sex (n)	Finger	Carpal	Finger	Carpal
Boys (26)	.845	.793	.881	.867
Girls (26)	.822	.780	.853	.842

be read in one sitting using the GP atlas, and the second file was of the same radiographs but in a different order, also to be read in one sitting using the GR atlas. Bone ages were recorded in years and months, and months were converted to the nearest tenth of a year. There was a high degree of correlation between readings done with the GP atlas and the readings of the same radiograph done with GR, with an ICC of 0.96. The mean reading of all bone ages was 9.22 by GP, and 9.26 by GR, indicating no trend for one atlas to give higher or lower bone age readings than the other.

The first edition of the electronic version of the digital atlas was developed for low resolution hand-held devices such as Palm Pilots and Pocket PC devices as well as a web-version for desktop computers. With this second edition a completely new digital application was developed for iPhone and iPad tablets. This second edition includes higher resolution images with a fully interactive user interface allowing continuous zoom and pan of the images.

Software User Manual

5

IPhone and IPad Apps

Software Installation

The software can be purchased and installed from the Apple App Store on the device or through the iTunes program. To know more about the App you can also check on the Springer Website at www.springer.com

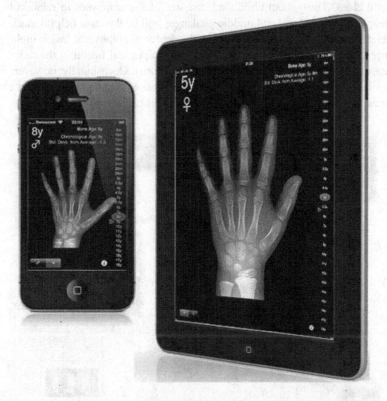

V. Gilsanz and O. Ratib, *Hand Bone Age*,
DOI 10.1007/978-3-642-23762-1_5, © Springer-Verlag Berlin Heidelberg 2012

Software User Manual

The App is designed to work on iPhone, iPod touch and iPad and will adapt to the
screen size with some minor differences in the user interface to better accommodate
the size and resolution of the screen. The user manual provided here is intended for
both platforms and will show different illustrations when the user interface differs
from one to another.

Starting the program: When launched the App will automatically display the
last image that was previously displayed (or the first one if it's the first time the app
is launched). On the right side of the screen you will find a vertical scale of ages.
The age corresponding to the image displayed is highlighted with a grey ellipse.
A yellow triangle shows the selected chronological age of the patient you are
examining. You can move both cursors independently.

Using the program: To estimate a patient's bone maturity from a hand radiograph
proceed as follows:

1. First, you must visually locate the image that best matches the hand and wrist
   radiograph to be interpreted. Browsing through images can be done either by moving the grey cursor along the age scale or by swiping the screen right and left. You
   should primarily focus on the centers that best characterize skeletal development
   for the subject's chronological age. During infancy and in toddlers, the presence or
   absence of certain carpal or epiphyseal ossification centers will provide the most
   useful clues. Throughout childhood, the size of the epiphyses in relation to the
   metaphysis in the distal and middle phalanges will be the most helpful markers of
   skeletal maturity. In younger teenagers, the degree of epiphyseal fusion in the phalanges, and in older teenagers, the degree of epiphyseal fusion in the radius and
   ulna, are the strongest indicators of skeletal maturity. Occasionally, however, there
   may be a disparity between the skeletal maturation of the phalanges and carpal
   bones. In such cases, two different estimated ages can be reported.

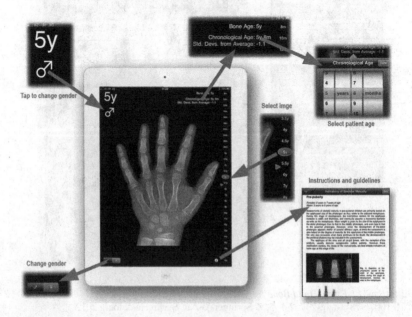

2. Once the matching image is identified, make sure to adjust the patient chronological age by moving the yellow triangle marker to its proper location on the age scale. You can also enter the patient's chronological age manually by taping on the displayed chronological age on the upper right corner of the image and a thumbwheel dialog will appear allowing you to select years and months to enter the patient's age. When done the standard deviation "SD" estimated from the difference between the selected bone age image and the actual chronological age of the patient is displayed on the second line below the patient's age.

3. You can also get help from the program by taping on the (i) button at the lower right corner of the screen. A short description of the specific findings to look for in the maturity range that is being explored will be displayed together with some explanatory illustrations.

Adjusting image display: you can zoom and pan each image using the standard "multi-touch" user interface of the iPhone or iPad. With two fingers you can zoom in and out of the image by pinching your fingers open and closed. With one finger you can move the image around the screen to locate a specific region of the hand. Double tapping with one finger on a given location of the image will automatically zoom in and out of the image with a magnification of 2×.

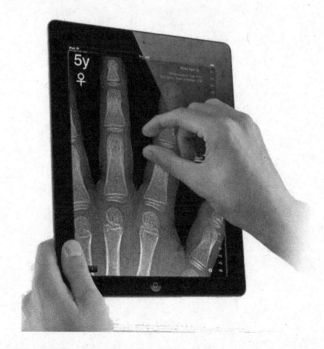

Selecting a gender: You can switch between boys and girls atlas simply by taping on the sex symbol on the upper left corner or on the gender switch in the lower left corner.

Reference Images

Caucasian Boys and Girls

V. Gilsanz and O. Ratib, *Hand Bone Age*,
DOI 10.1007/978-3-642-23762-1_6, © Springer-Verlag Berlin Heidelberg 2012

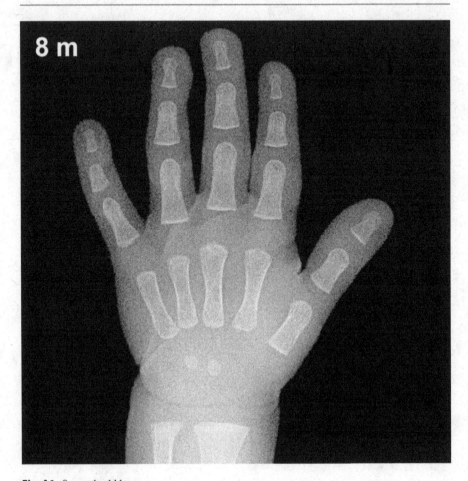

Fig. A1 8-month-old boy

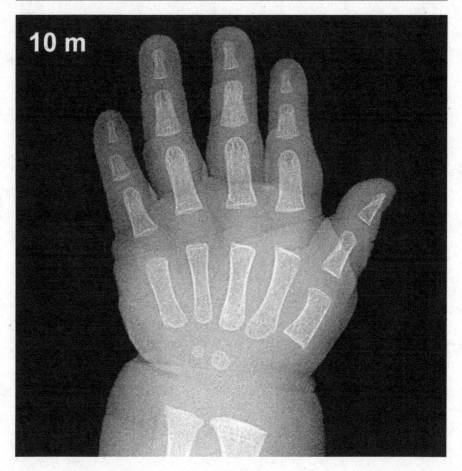

Fig. A2 10-month-old boy

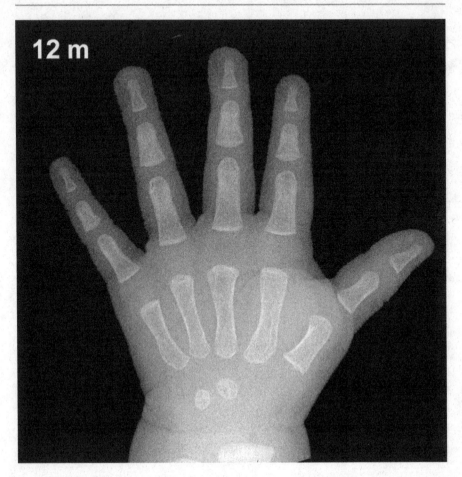

Fig. A3 12-month-old boy

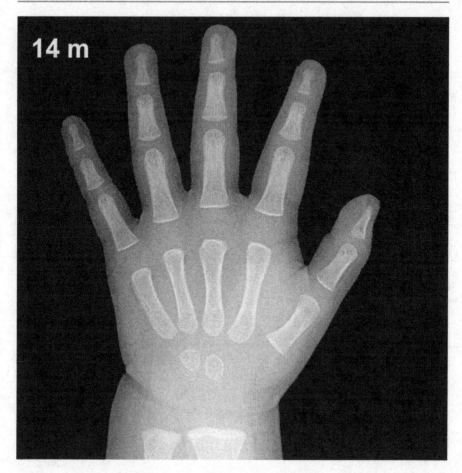

Fig. A4 14-month-old boy

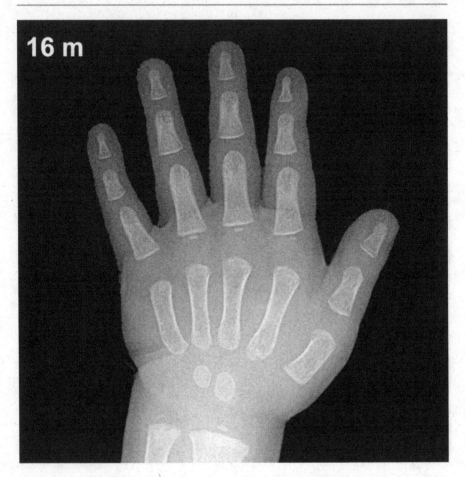

16 m

Fig. A5 16-month-old boy

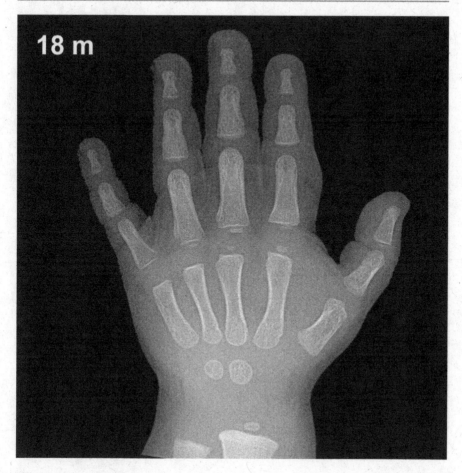

Fig. A6 18-month-old boy

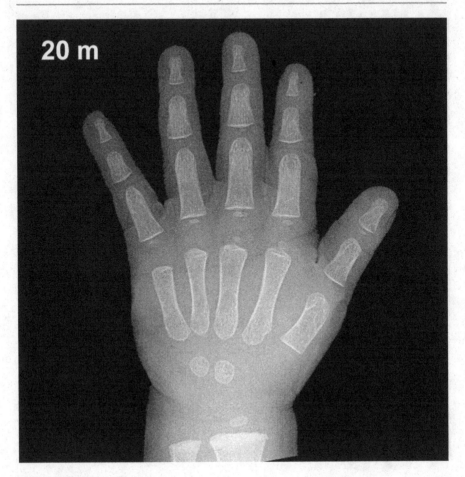

Fig. A7 20-month-old boy

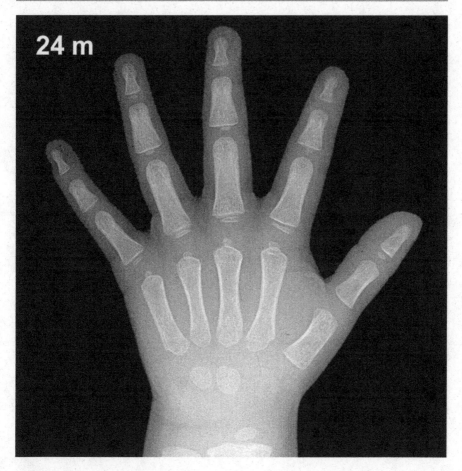

Fig. A8 2-year-old boy

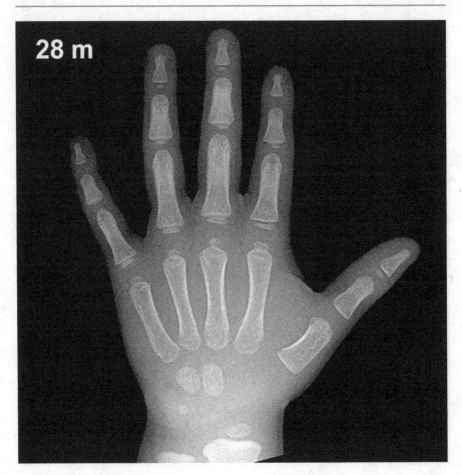

Fig. A9   28-month-old boy

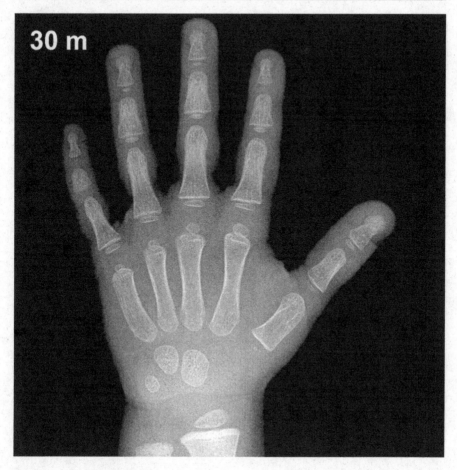

Fig. A10   2.5-year-old boy

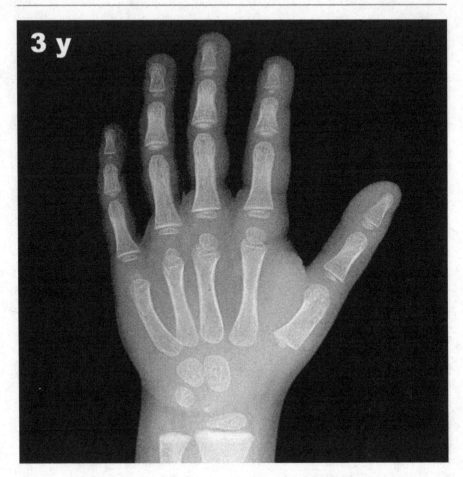

Fig. A11 3-year-old boy

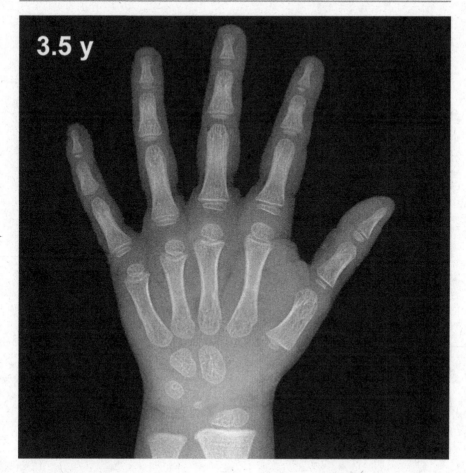

Fig. A12 3.5-year-old boy

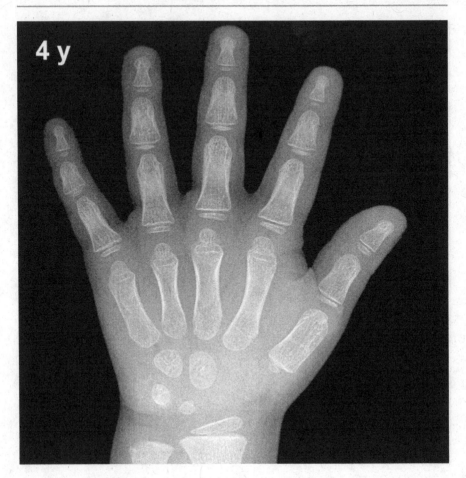

Fig. A13 4-year-old boy

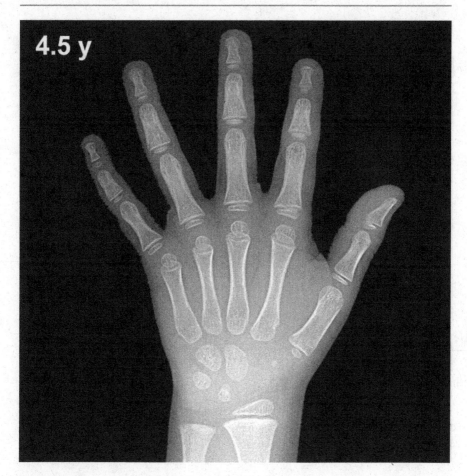

Fig. A14   4.5-year-old boy

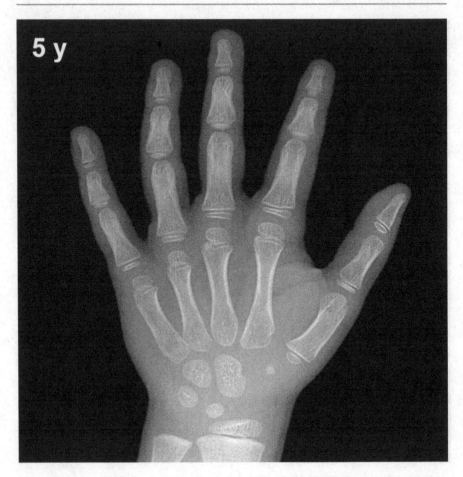

Fig. A15 5-year-old boy

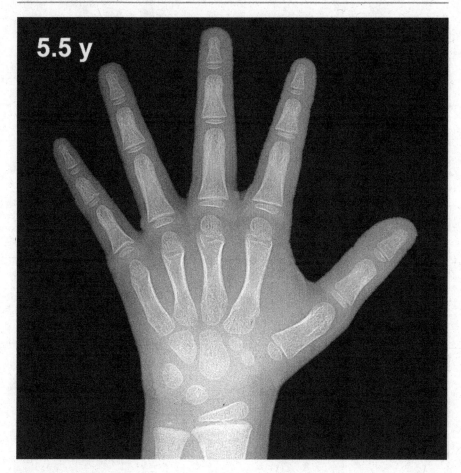

Fig. A16 5.5-year-old boy

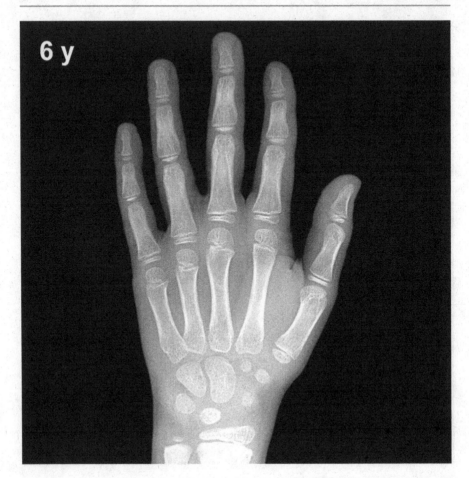

6 y

Fig. A17 6-year-old boy

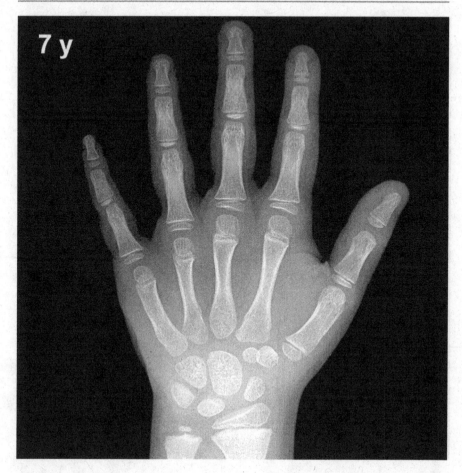

Fig. A18 7-year-old boy

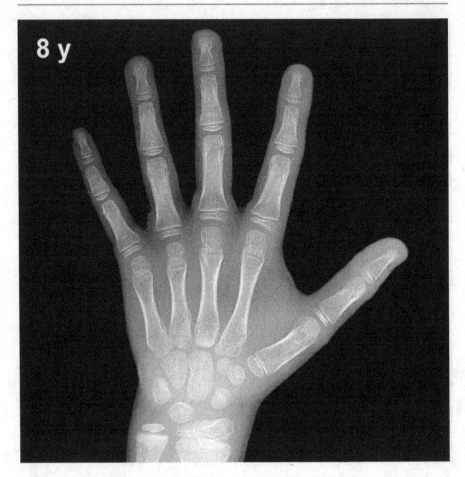

8 y

Fig. A19 8-year-old boy

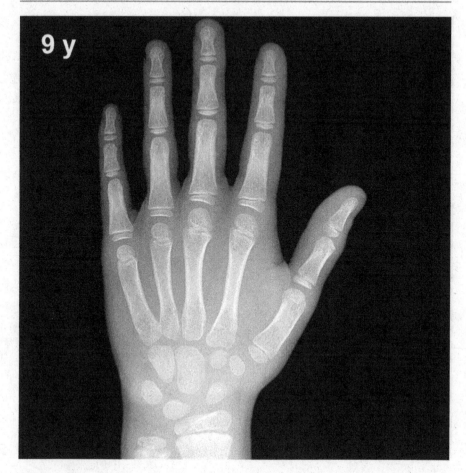

Fig. A20 9-year-old boy

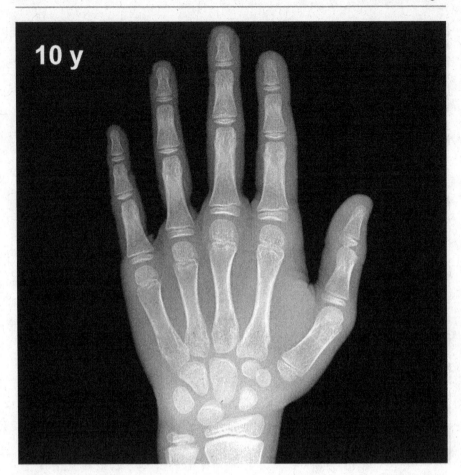

Fig. A21   10-year-old boy

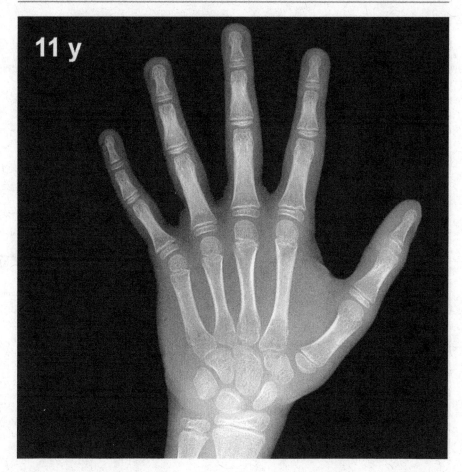

Fig. A22 11-year-old boy

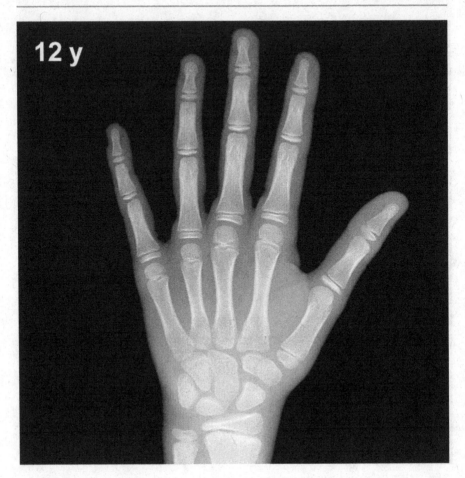

Fig. A23   12-year-old boy

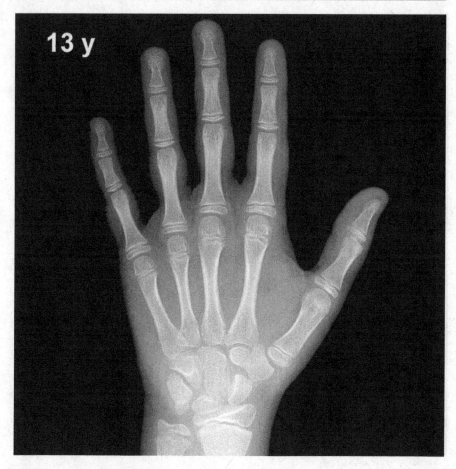

Fig. A24 13-year-old boy

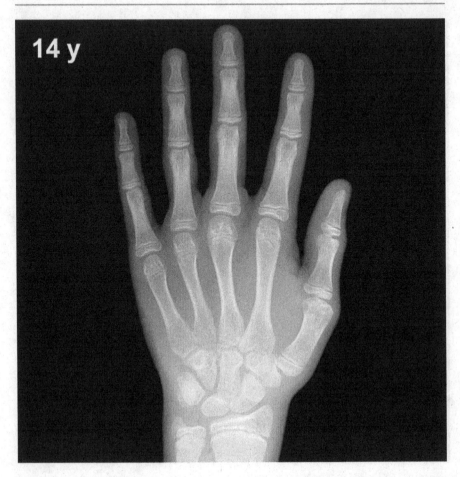

14 y

Fig. A25 14-year-old boy

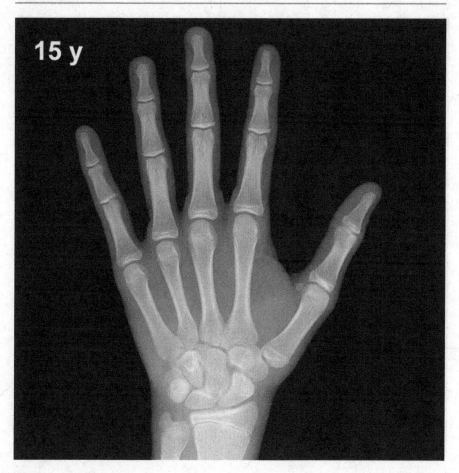

Fig. A26   15-year-old boy

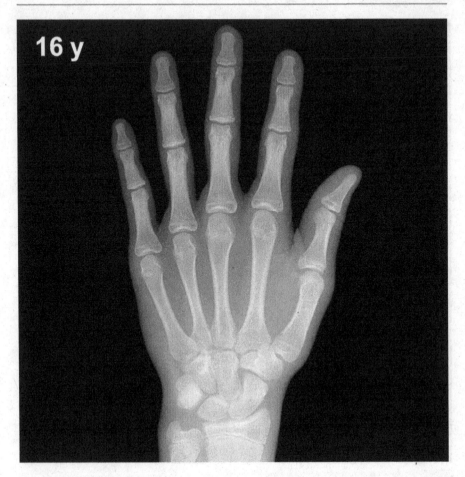

Fig. A27   16-year-old boy

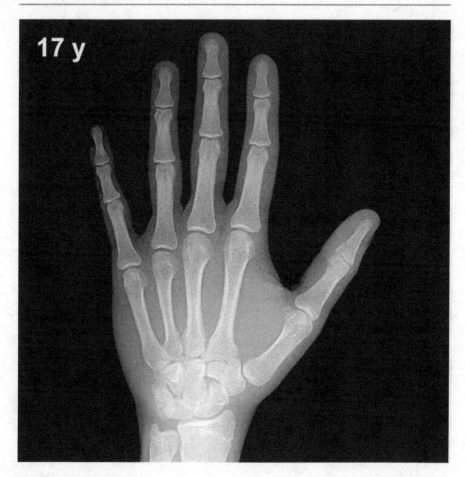

Fig. A28   17-year-old boy

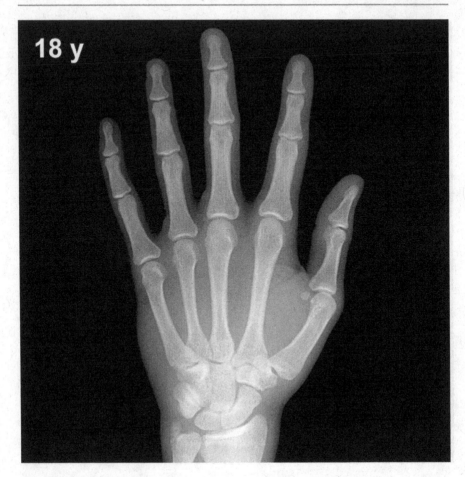

18 y

Fig. A29 18-year-old boy

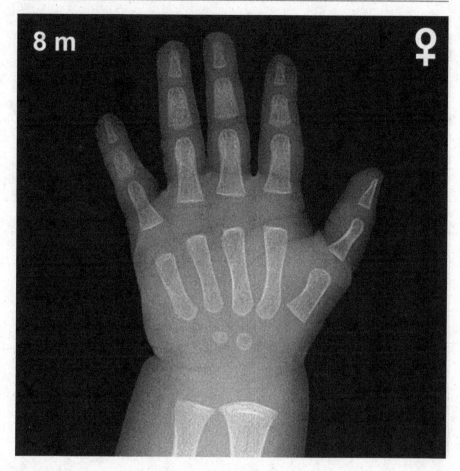

Fig. A30 8-month-old girl

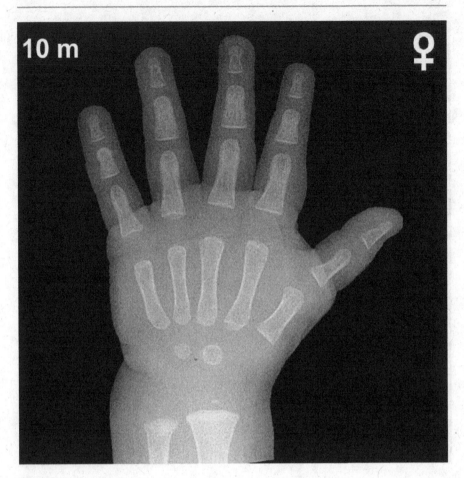

Fig. A31 10-month-old girl

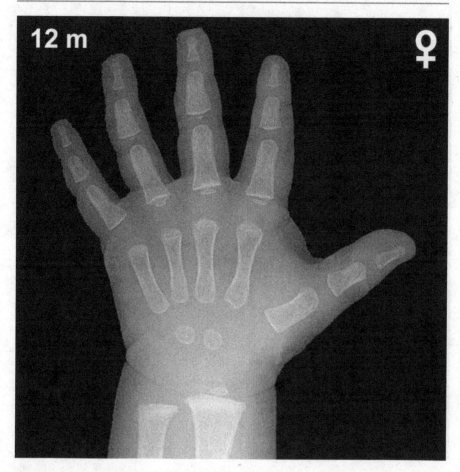

Fig. A32 12-month-old girl

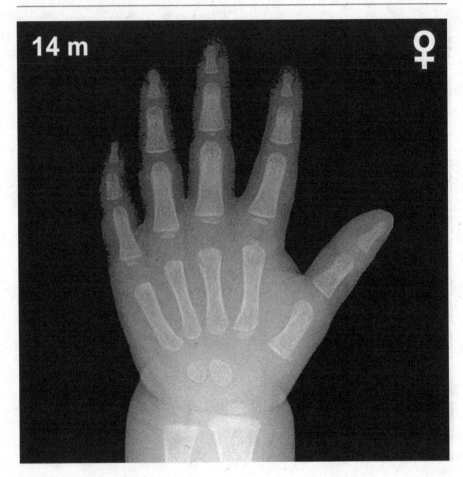

Fig. A33 14-month-old girl

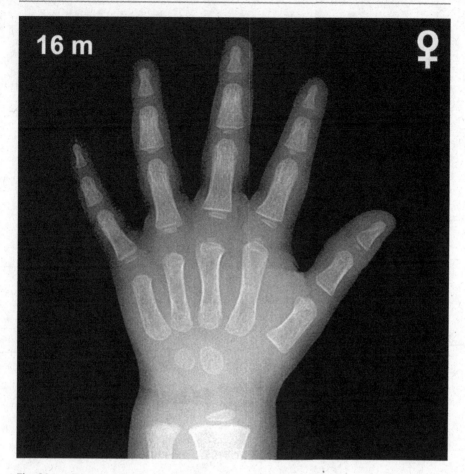

Fig. A34 16-month-old girl

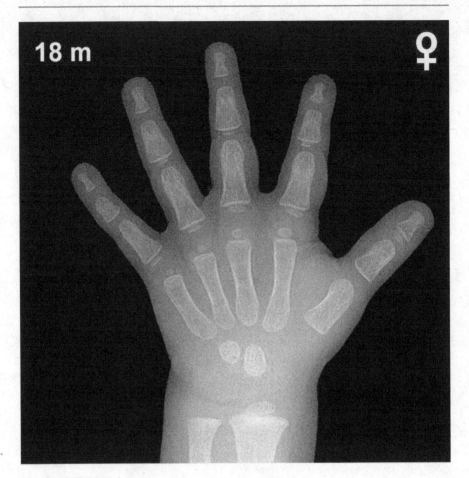

Fig. A35 18-month-old girl

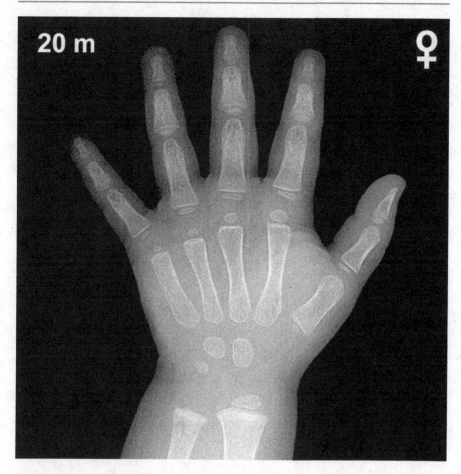

20 m

Fig. A36 20-month-old girl

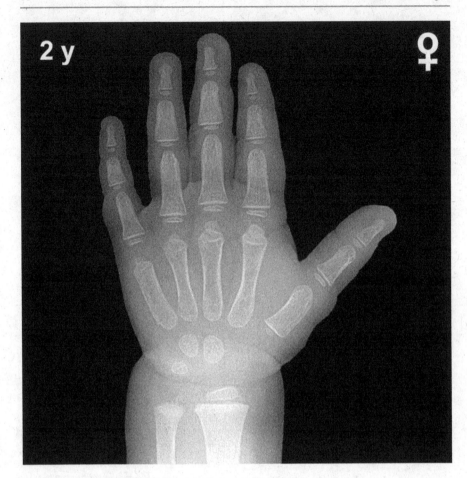

Fig. A37 24-month-old girl

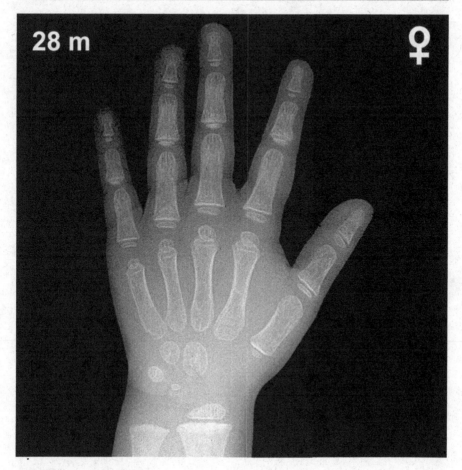

Fig. A38   28-month-old girl

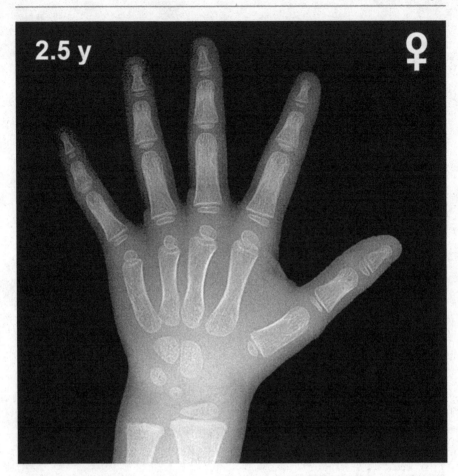

Fig. A39   2.5-year-old girl

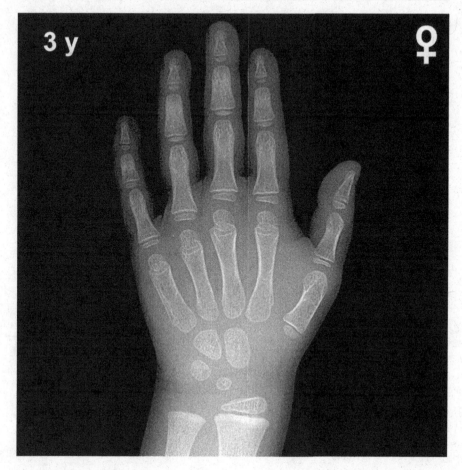

Fig. A40 3-year-old girl

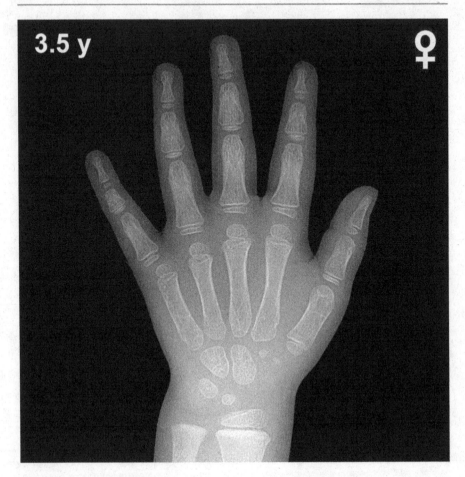

Fig. A41 3.5-year-old girl

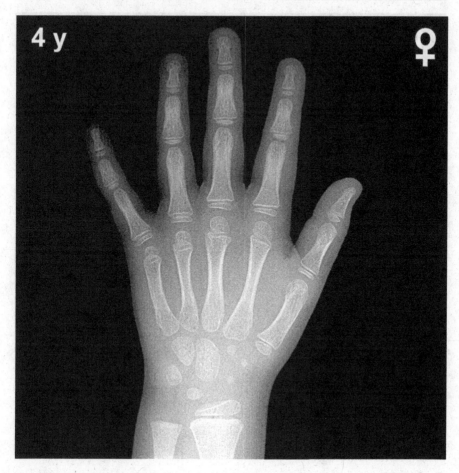

Fig. A42 4-year-old girl

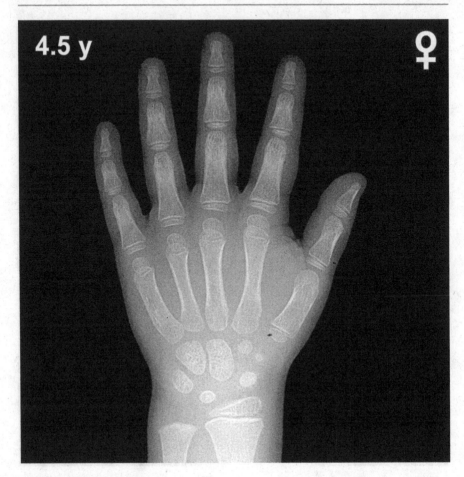

Fig. A43 4.5-year-old girl

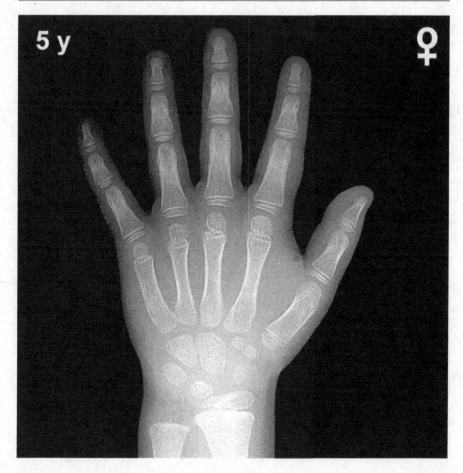

Fig. A44 5-year-old girl

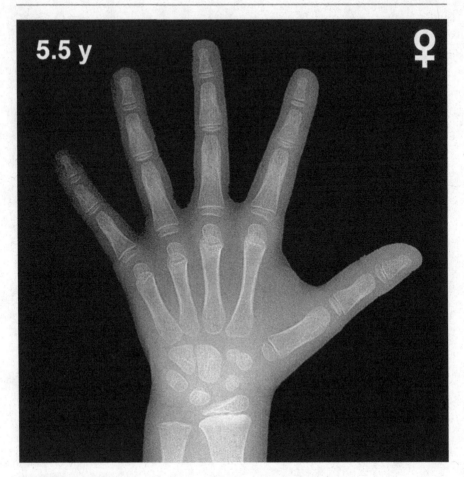

5.5 y

♀

Fig. A45   5.5-year-old girl

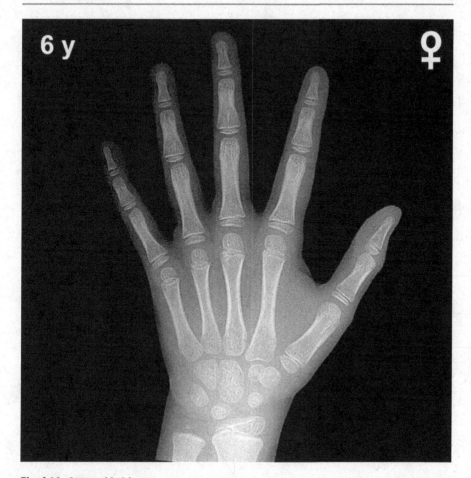

Fig. A46 6-year-old girl

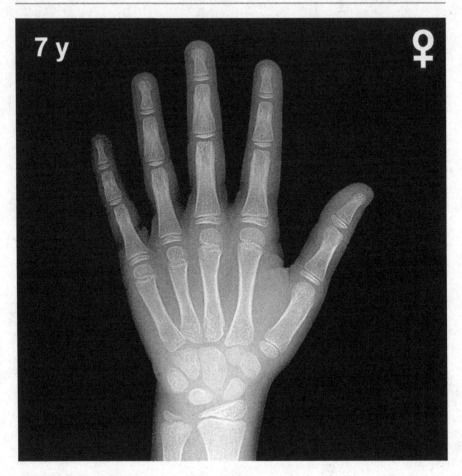

Fig. A47 7-year-old girl

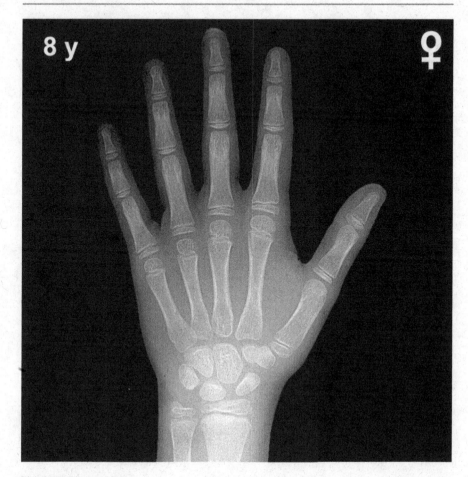

Fig. A48 8-year-old girl

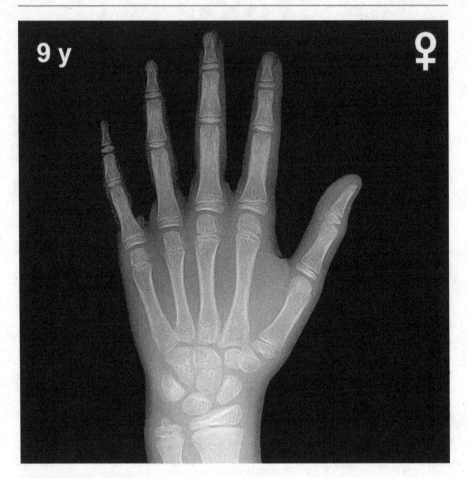

Fig. A49 9-year-old girl

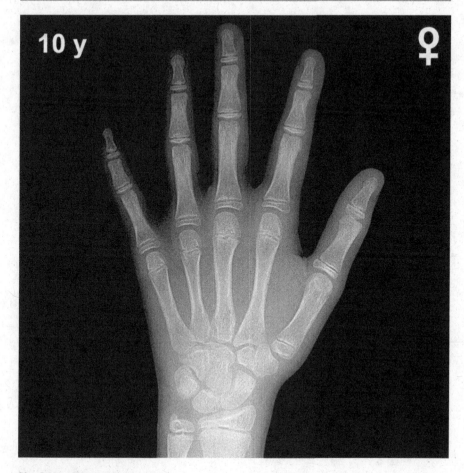

Fig. A50 10-year-old girl

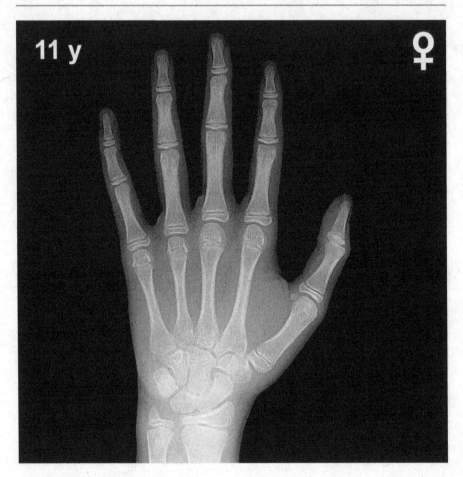

Fig. A51 11-year-old girl

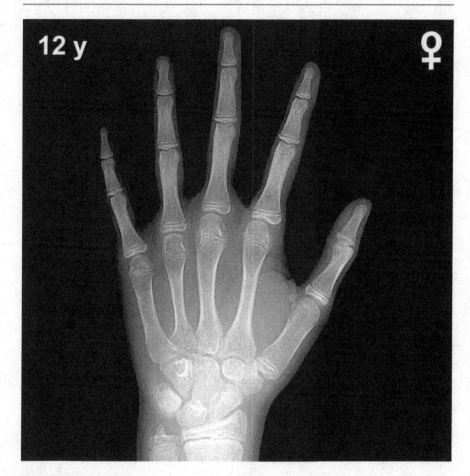

Fig. A52 12-year-old girl

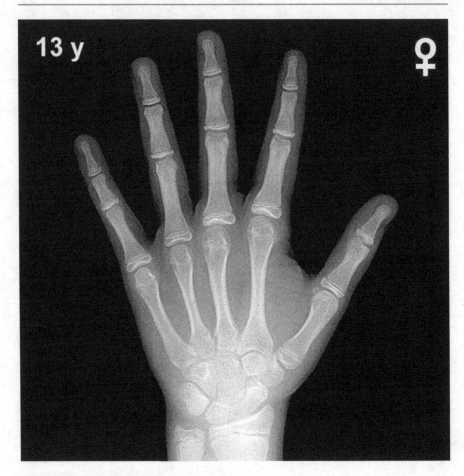

Fig. A53 13-year-old girl

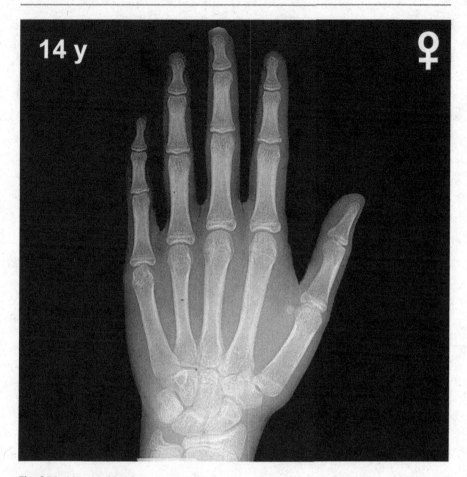

14 y

Fig. A54 14-year-old girl

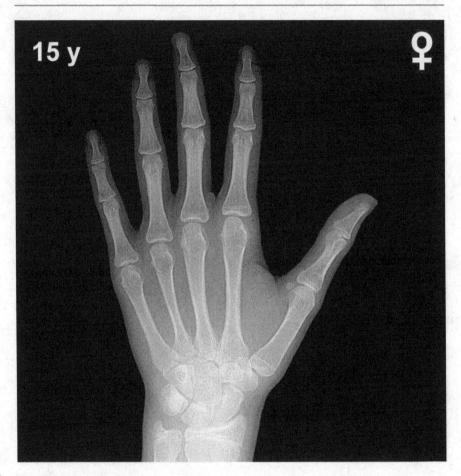

Fig. A55 15-year-old girl

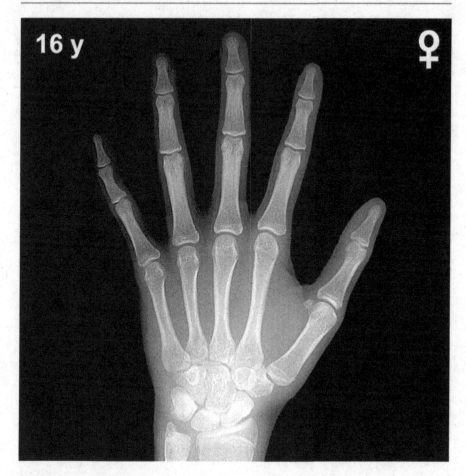

Fig. A56 16-year-old girl

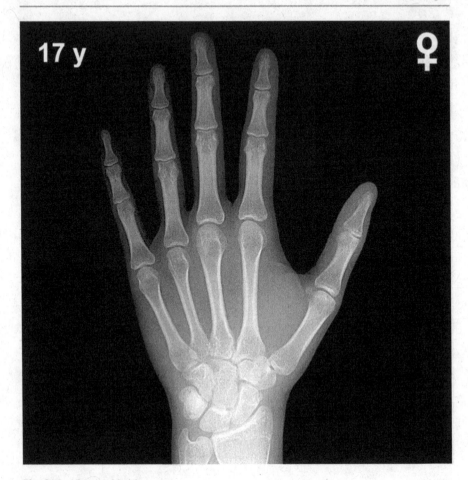

Fig. A57 17-year-old girl

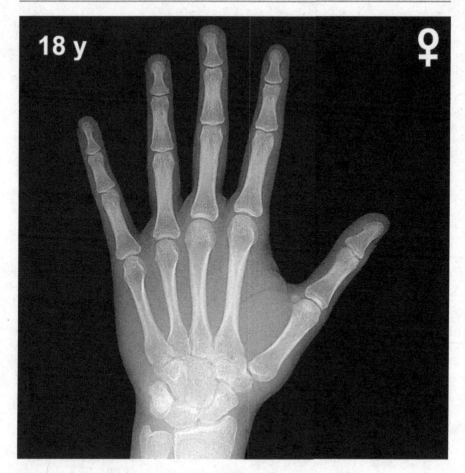

Fig. A58 18-year-old girl

Tables

Table 7.1 Coefficients for prediction of adult height for boys

Age (years)	Coefficient for height	Coefficient for age	Coefficient for bone age	Constant
4–7	1.20	−7.3	0	82
8.0	1.22	−7.2	−0.4	82
8.5	1.23	−7.0	−0.7	82
9.0	1.22	−6.8	−0.8	82
9.5	1.21	−6.5	−0.8	82
10.0	1.20	−6.2	−1.0	83
10.5	1.19	−5.9	−1.2	84
11.0	1.16	−5.5	−1.6	89
11.5	1.13	−5.1	−2.0	94
12.0	1.08	−4.2	−2.6	98
12.5	1.03	−3.4	−3.2	108
13.0	0.98	−2.6	−3.8	108
13.5	0.94	−1.9	−4.4	113
14.0	0.90	−1.4	−4.5	114
14.5	0.87	−1.0	−4.6	114
15.0	0.84	−0.8	−3.8	104
15.5	0.82	−0.6	−3.1	94
16.0	0.88	−0.4	−2.4	71
16.5	0.94	−0.3	−1.8	48
17.0	0.96	−0.2	−1.2	34
17.5	0.98	−0.1	−0.7	19

Adapted from reference [9]

V. Gilsanz and O. Ratib, *Hand Bone Age*,
DOI 10.1007/978-3-642-23762-1_7, © Springer-Verlag Berlin Heidelberg 2012

Example

A boy is referred because his parents are worried about his short stature. He is 13.5 years old and 145 cm in height, corresponding to the 3rd percentile. His bone age is determined to be 12 years. From Table 7.1 we can obtain his predicted final height:
$(0.94 \times 145) + (-1.9 \times 13.5) + (-4.4 \times 12) + 113 = 136.3 - 25.65 - 52.8 + 113$
$= 170.85$ cm.

Table 7.2 Coefficients for prediction of adult height for girls

Age (years)	Coefficient for height	Coefficient for age	Coefficient for bone age	Constant
Premenarche				
4–5	0.95	−6.5	0	93
6.0	0.95	−6.0	−0.4	93
6.5	0.95	−5.5	−0.8	93
7.0	0.94	−5.1	−1.0	94
7.5	0.93	−4.7	−1.1	94
8.0	0.92	−4.4	−1.5	95
8.5	0.92	−4.0	−1.9	96
9.0	0.92	−3.8	−2.3	99
9.5	0.91	−3.6	−2.7	102
10.0	0.89	−3.2	−3.2	106
10.5	0.87	−2.7	−3.6	109
11.0	0.83	−2.6	−3.6	114
11.5	0.82	−2.5	−3.6	115
12.0	0.83	−2.4	−3.4	111
12.5	0.83	−2.3	−3.3	108
13.0	0.85	−2.0	−3.1	98
13.5	0.87	−1.8	−3.0	90
14.0	0.91	−1.6	−2.8	79
14.5	0.99	−1.4	−2.5	67
Postmenarche				
11.0	0.87	−2.3	−3.3	100
11.5	0.89	−1.9	−3.3	91
12.0	0.91	−1.4	−3.2	82
12.5	0.93	−1.0	−2.7	67
13.0	0.95	−0.9	−2.2	55
13.5	0.96	−0.9	−1.8	48
14.0	0.96	−0.8	−1.4	40
14.5	0.97	−0.8	−1.3	37
15.0	0.98	−0.6	−1.1	30
15.5	0.99	−0.4	−0.7	20

Adapted from reference [9]

Example

A girl is referred because she is worried she will be too tall when she grows up. She is 11 years old and 158 cm in height, about the 97th percentile. Her bone age is determined to be 12, and she is premenarche. From Table 7.2 we can obtain her predicted final height: $(0.83 \times 158) + (-2.2 \times 11) + (-3.6 \times 12) + 114 = 131.14 - 24.2 - 43.2 + 114 = 177.74$ cm.

The standard deviation calculation for each age category in the digital bone age atlas was based on the equation for the linear regression that best fit the variability of multiple samples at different ages.

Table 7.3 Tanner stages of sexual development

Females		Male	
Stage	Mean age (years ± SD)	Stage	Mean age (years ± SD)
Breast 2	11.2 ± 1.1	Genital 2	11.4 ± 1.1
Pubic hair 2	11.7 ± 1.2	Pubic hair 2	12.0 ± 1.0
Breast 3	12.2 ± 1.1	Genital 3	12.9 ± 1.0
Pubic hair 3	12.4 ± 1.1	Pubic hair 3	13.9 ± 1.0
Breast 4	13.1 ± 1.2	Genital 4	13.8 ± 1.0
Pubic hair 4	13.0 ± 1.1	Pubic hair 4	14.4 ± 1.1
Breast 5	15.3 ± 1.7	Genital 5	14.9 ± 1.1
Pubic hair 5	14.4 ± 1.1	Pubic hair 5	15.2 ± 1.1
Menarche	13.5 ± 1.0	–	–

Adapted from references [19, 20]

Table 7.4 Variability in bone age

Age in months	Boys SD	Girls SD
12	2.1	2.7
18	2.7	3.4
24	4	4
30	5.4	4.8
36	6	5.6
42	6.6	5.5
48	7	7.2
54	7.8	8
60	8.4	8.6
66	9.1	8.9
72	9.3	9
84	10.1	8.3
96	10.8	8.8
108	11	9.3
120	11.4	10.8
132	10.5	12.3
144	10.4	14
156	11.1	14.6
168	12	12.6
180	14	11.2
192	15	15
204	15.4	15.4

References

1. Lowrey GH (1986) Growth and development of children, 8th edn. Year Book Medical Publishers, Inc., Chicago
2. Kuhns LR, Finnstrom O (1976) New standards of ossification of the newborn. Radiology 119:655–660
3. Keats TE (2004) The bones: normal and variants. In: Kuhn JP, Slovis TL, Haller JO (eds) Caffey's pediatric diagnostic imaging, 10th edn. Mosby, Philadelphia, pp 2035–2092
4. Morishima A, Gumbach MM, Simpson ER, Fisher C, Qin K (1995) Aromatase deficiency in male and female siblings caused by a novel mutation and the physiological role of estrogens. J Clin Endocrinol Metab 80:3689–3698
5. Kaplan SA (1990) Growth and growth hormone: disorders of the anterior pituitary. In: Kaplan SA (ed) Clinical pediatric endocrinology, 2nd edn. W. B. Saunders Company, Philadelphia, pp 1–62
6. Rosenfeld RG, Cohen P (2002) Disorders of growth hormone/insulin-like growth factor secretion and action. In: Sperling MA (ed) Pediatric endocrinology. Saunders, Philadelphia, pp 211–288
7. Bayley N, Pinneau SR (1952) Tables for predicting adult height from skeletal age: revised for use with Greulich-Pyle hand standards. J Pediatr 40:423
8. Roche AF, Wainer H, Thissen D (1975) The RWT method for the prediction of adult stature. Pediatrics 56:1026
9. Tanner JM, Whitehouse RH, Marshall WA et al (1975) Prediction of adult height from height, bone age, and occurrence of menarche at ages 4–16 with allowance for midparent height. Arch Dis Child 50:14
10. Greulich WW, Pyle SI (1959) Radiographic atlas of skeletal development of the hand and wrist, 2nd edn. Stanford University Press, California
11. Tanner JM, Whitehouse RH, Marshall WA et al (1975) Assessment of skeletal maturity and prediction of adult height (TW2 Method). Academic Press, New York
12. Roche AF, Davila GH, Eyman SL (1971) A comparison between Greulich-Pyle and Tanner-Whitehouse assessments of skeletal maturity. Radiology 98:273
13. Tanner JM, Gibbons RD (1994) A computerized image analysis system for estimating Tanner-Whitehouse 2 bone age. Horm Res 42:282–287
14. Tanner JM, Oshman D, Lindgren G, Grunbaum JA, Elsouki R, Labarthe DR (1994) Reliability and validity of computer-assisted estimates of Tanner-Whitehouse skeletal maturity (CASAS): comparison with the manual method. Horm Res 42:288–294
15. Dickhaus H, Wastl S (1995) Computer assisted bone age assessment. Medinfo 8:709–713
16. Cao F, Huang HK, Pietka E, Gilsanz V (2000) Digital hand atlas and web-based bone age assessment: system design and implementation. Comput Med Imaging Graph 24:297–307

17. Pietka E, Pospiech S, Gertych A, Cao F, Huang HK, Gilsanz V (2001) Computer automated approach to the extraction of epiphyseal regions in hand radiographs. J Digit Imaging 14: 165–172
18. Garn SM, Rohmann CG, Silverman FN (1967) Radiographic standards for postnatal ossification and tooth calcification. Med Radiogr Photogr 43:45–66
19. Marshall WA, Tanner JM (1970) Variations in the pattern of pubertal changes in boys. Arch Dis Child 45:13
20. Marshall WA, Tanner JM (1969) Variations in the pattern of pubertal changes in girls. Arch Dis Child 44:291
21. Kaplowitz P, Srinivasan S, He J, McCarter R, Hayeri MR, Sze R (2011) Comparison of bone age readings by pediatric endocrinologists and pediatric radiologists using two bone age atlases. Pediatr Radiol 41:690–693